Homemade Repellents:

25 Non-Toxic Recipes To Keep Away Mosquitoes

Table of content

Introduction

If you're reading this book, you may already know the answer, but for many people, there is a question of why one needs to make a homemade repellent. The short answer is that there are many reasons. For some, it's an issue of reducing the amount of synthetic pesticides and chemicals. For others it's more of an issue of being prepared for any circumstance. Regardless of the reason, no one likes being eaten alive by mosquitoes, and in the modern world of bug resistance repellents and insects that carry everything from Zika to chikungunya and dengue fever, which is spreading across the industrialized world, warding off mosquitoes is more than just a desire; it's an absolute necessity.

If your goal is to get closer to nature, one of the down sides of that life is that you often do things or carry out tasks that are likely to attract more mosquitoes. Whether it's composting, farming, hiking, or gardening, mosquitoes are often not far behind. The good news is that you don't have to take it lying down any longer.

This book will lay out 25 easy do it yourself recipes that you'll be able to make and adjust as needed. The great thing about many of these recipes is that you don't need a lab or special ingredients. You can use basic ingredients from just about any grocery, supply, or hobby store. As a bonus, you'll also find several tricks, tips, and suggestions to help you along the way. In addition, we will analyze the effectiveness for certain common ingredients and suggested tips so that you can have all the facts before you lay out your plan to ward off these nasty pests.

Chapter 1 – Tips & Tricks

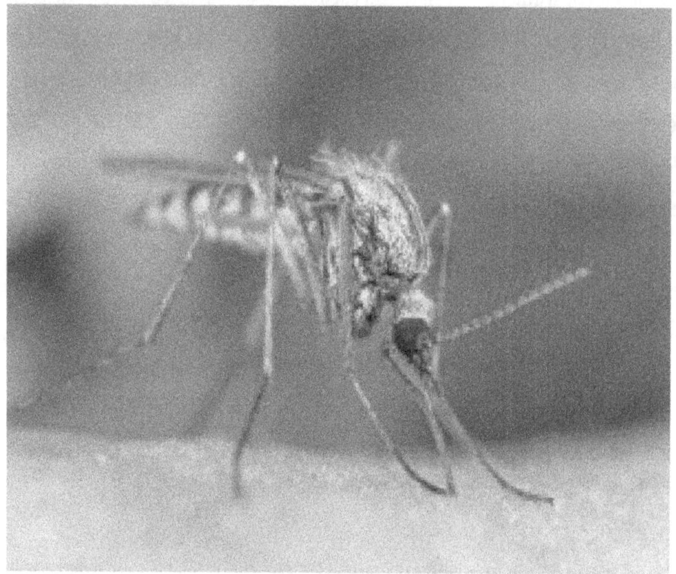

Before you get started on making your repellent, don't forget that the same rules to avoiding mosquitoes still apply. If you are going to a place where you know there is a lot of mosquitoes, cover your skin. Wear long pants and shirts, if at all possible, and keep your socks tucked over your pants. In addition, make sure that you wash regularly. Mosquitoes are attracted to lactic acid, which is a byproduct of exercise. Being hot and sweaty tends to attract more mosquitoes, so stay cool and stay dry.

Another common misconception about mosquitoes is that they are attracted to certain colors. It has been said that mosquitoes are more attracted to dark colors, with a preference for blue. According to the CDC, there is no evidence to support the claim, so don't throw away your dark colored clothes or blue jeans just yet. While a study from the Caltech did show dark colors attracted the insects, there was a caveat. Mosquitoes only use color to hone in on a target once they've located a carbon dioxide plume and movement. Switching to a lighter color of clothing won't provide you additional protection. Mosquitoes are attracted to specific things such as carbon dioxide, heat, and movement. Changing colors will do little to protect you once your breath has been spotted.

Mosquito nets are still recommended for malaria infested regions, so don't chuck all the safety precautions just because you have some repellent. If you do so, you only heighten your risk of getting eaten. Of course, we all can't wear long pants and sleeves all the time, but you should still take measures wherever possible to limit skin exposure. Mosquitoes also are more attractive to adults over children and men over women because of the size. but that doesn't mean you are safe just because you're are female or under the age of eighteen.

With respect to the actual ingredients with DIY repellent, it's important to look at some science before we get into the actual recipes. This is extremely important because some things work better than others, and some things don't work at all. There are a few classes of plants, though, that we can target and include in the home recipes.

The good news is that there is some testing by agencies that compared synthetic chemicals such as DEET and PMD to ingredients such as certain essential oils. DEET is the most effective in terms of strength and duration, but that is when comparing it to the same concentrations of other options. Adding higher concentrations of the alternative ingredients may still provide some protection. In the article referenced above, maintaining a concentration of the essential oils at 20% can retain the effectiveness of homemade repellent close to 90% for 5 hours. At the 10% level, the oils held up at about 80% effective for up to five hours. As such, it is recommended your recipes contain at least 10% of one of the tested essential oils.

Any of the recipes listed here or elsewhere can be modified by adding 11% to 22% of a tested essential oil by weight or mass to the original recipe's final product before adding the oil. Without adding a known tested ingredient, such as an essential oil, it really is just a crap shoot on whether or not your repellent will be effective. As such, it's recommended sure that your recipe includes it, if not, add it after the fact. Otherwise, you have no guarantee that your recipe will do what it's intended to do and might even cause more harm than good.

Mosquitoes are attracted to certain scents, so if your recipe smells good but has no active ingredient to ward them off, you may actually be attracting mosquitoes instead of repelling them. Keep in mind, though, that not all oils are created equally. A popular oil is citronella, but again, the CDC has stated that citronella oil is a very weak repellent, and the candles likely only protect the candle.

One specific oil, which was studied by the American Chemical Society and reported by Science News Daily.

I would also caution against supplements. Some have suggested taking vitamin B1 (Thiamin) or other supplements can help keep away mosquitoes. There is little evidence to support this theory, so I recommend against it. Supplements can also interact with certain medications, so think twice before you try that approach and consult with your doctor regarding any medications you are currently taking. Changing your diet, whether adding or removing certain foods, will have little impact on the chances of being bitten. That goes for garlic as well. It has no impact, none.

You may also have read that having O type blood increases your odds of being attacked, along with drinking beer. Again, the evidence does not support that. Feel free to drink beer without getting attacked, and your blood type has no bearing on the likelihood of getting bitten. That was simply a case of a bad study with bad statistics.

When it comes to attracting the female mosquitoes that bite, it really comes down to limiting your exposure and making your skin less attractive. What makes you attractive to the female mosquitoes in the first place is a combination of carbon dioxide and certain scents, scents that alert the mosquitoes to fats, lactic acid, and sugars in your blood. Whether you are using essential oils, or chemicals such as DEET, they target the same mechanism.

As discussed by ABC in a recent segment, scents are the magnets, and masking those scents is how repellents work. Evidence shows that smelly feet, and scented deodorants attract mosquitoes. Smelly or overly sweet creams or sprays, including perfumes, will also attract mosquitoes. The remedy that, stay clean and use unscented perfumes and creams as much as possible. The smell from essential oils are likely what wards off the mosquitoes in the first place, and if you add other scents they are attracted to, you may lessen the effectiveness of those repellents.

As a general rule, you want to avoid adding or switching additional untested ingredients that are noticeably strong or sweet. If you are using certain things such as processed aloe vera or other filler or secondary ingredients in modified recipes, opt for those that are unscented or have the least amount of scent.

If you've already been bitten, don't scratch! Rub gently with a flat finger if you have too, but do not scratch. Scratching introducing bacteria and increases the chance for infection and lengthens the time needed for healing. If you don't feel comfortable using antihistamine creams for bites, use ice instead. Ice can be just as effective.

Another strategy is to add creams or ingredients within your repellent that sooths skin. Again, make sure you avoid scented varieties, but adding a moisturizer or other ingredient such as aloe vera is a great way to aid healing while at the same time protecting your skin.

Chapter 2 – Clearing The Yard

With a little research, along with your new knowledge of certain plants and essential oils, you can do certain things to reduce the amount of mosquitoes in your yard and in your home before you even start making sprays.

A few sites have recommended using bats as a mosquito deterrent. While that may be effective, you're also likely to dramatically increase your risk of contracting rabies. Bat bites just happen to be the single biggest cause of rabies in humans according to the CDC, so I wouldn't recommend it.

In your home and on your property, make sure that you keep it dry and clean. Clear any standing leaves, debris, or water. Debris can hold pockets of water and keep the ground damp and moist, which is a breeding ground for mosquitoes. You should also keep your lawn mowed and trim hedges and weeds. A well maintained lawn and yard will minimize the opportunity for insects.

Once you've cleaned your lawn, double check any standing structure, which can be anything from a toy to a lawn gnome. Even well maintained yards can have pockets of standing water in hidden places, so make sure your check is thorough. You should also keep all food covered with lids, and tighten any existing lids. This help limit standing water and limits hiding places of mosquitoes.

Once you've done the heavy lifting, you may be tempted by citronella candles or smoking coils. Both of these are only effective when people are completely covered in the smoke plume. In other words, they are worthless. One study even showed that if a person had the smoke plume covering he top of the leg, mosquitoes bit the bottom half! No one is going to be fully covered in a smoke plume. Save your money.

Another thing you can do to reduce your yards attractiveness to mosquitoes is by getting rid of candlelight and ultra-violent lighting. These types of lights have been shown to attract the mosquitoes, so eliminate both of these to reduce their frequency. Some bug zappers use ultra-violent lighting. They are only minimally effective at killing the mosquitoes, but end up attracting them, increasing the likelihood they the newly attracted mosquitoes find a water source to lay their eggs, breeding even more mosquitoes. Again, save your money.

Planting a garden with specific plants, or even the plants that are used in making the essential oils, is a common suggestion by many sites, giving advice on how to limit mosquitoes. While, these plants likely won't attract more mosquitoes, any protection provided by the plants would be minimal and primarily protect the plant itself. If you still want to plant them, have at it, just understand that you will have little or no extra protection on your person.

Chapter 3 – Recipes 1-8 Sichuan Pepper (Zanthoxylum limonella)

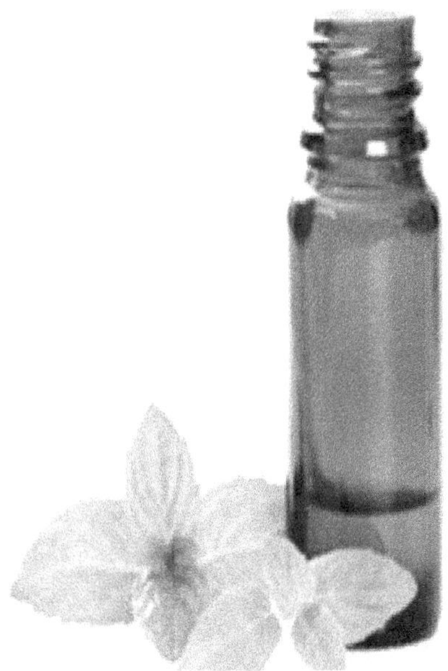

Before using any of the recipes listed in the next few chapters, make sure that you do not have allergic reactions to any of the ingredients. Many people don't often come in contact with essential oils or base oils in high concentrations, so ask a doctor or test a small sample area with a lower concentration first if you are unsure.

The first four recipes are going to be your most effective. If you only make four recipes, use these four. The article referenced in the earlier chapter showed that the essential oil of Sichuan pepper was the most effective essential oil tested. You can find 7 oz bottles for about $15-$20, and you don't need to use the whole bottle.

In addition, there is a base of mustard oil that you can use with the Sichuan. Coconut oil can also be replaced by mustard oil, but is slightly less effective. Below are eight different recipes that use either mustard oil or coconut oil. Outside of the two main ingredients, the base and the essential oil, all of it can be modified or changed without much difficulty. Just keep in mind that mosquitoes are attracted to scent, sweet and smelly scents in particular.

Recipe #1: The first recipe is the basic and simple. Use one ounce of 100% Sichuan Pepper (Zanthoxylum limonella) oil and four ounces of 100% Mustard oil as a base. This will yield 5 ounces of repellent, and should be enough for several applications. This recipe is a 20% essential oil solution in the most effective base with no extra fillers. The cost for this recipe is around $3; that's $2 for the one ounce of Sichuan, and $1 for the mustard oil.

Recipe #2: This recipe adds aloe vera, and will reduce the smelliness of the mustard oil while adding additional healing properties to the skin. Use one ounce of 100% Sichuan Pepper (Zanthoxylum limonella) oil, two ounces of 100% Mustard oil as a base, and two ounces of aloe vera gel. The aloe vera gel can be in any form you wish, whether its straight from the plant or from a processed cream or gel from the store. This will also yield 5 ounces of repellent for several applications and cost around the same price as the first recipe. As mentioned earlier, select a version of aloe vera gel that is unscented or has as little scent as possible to maintain the effectiveness of the Sichuan.

Recipe #3: This recipe adds aloe vera and is very similar to recipe #2. It still uses mustard oil, but the aloe vera is used in greater proportion to further mask the smell. Use one ounce of 100% Sichuan Pepper (Zanthoxylum limonella) oil, one ounce of 100% Mustard oil as a base, and three ounces of aloe vera gel. The price point is around $3, as in the recipe #2.

Recipe #4: This recipe eliminates the mustard oil completely as is a good option for those with reactions to mustard oil or for those who hate the scent or feel of the mustard oil. It still uses 20% Sichuan, but the removal of the mustard oil will likely reduce the duration of its protection. Use one ounce of 100% Sichuan Pepper (Zanthoxylum limonella) oil, four ounces of aloe vera gel. The price point is around $3, that's $2 for the Sichuan and $1 for the aloe vera.

Recipe #5: This recipe is uses one ounce of 100% Sichuan Pepper (Zanthoxylum limonella) oil and four ounces of 100% coconut oil as a base. This will yield 5 ounces of repellent, and should be enough for several applications. This recipe is a 20% essential oil solution in an effective base with no extra fillers, though not quite as effective as the mustard oil base options. The cost for this recipe is around $3; that's $2 for the one ounce of Sichuan, and $1 for the coconut oil.

Recipe #6: This recipe adds aloe vera, and will reduce the adding additional healing properties to the skin by using both aloe vera gel and coconut oil. Use one ounce of 100% Sichuan Pepper (Zanthoxylum limonella) oil, two ounces of 100% coconut oil as a base, and two ounces of aloe vera gel. The cost for this recipe is around $3; that's $2 for the one ounce of Sichuan, and $1 for the coconut oil.

Recipe #7: This recipe is similar to #6 but uses more aloe vera gel. Use one ounce of 100% Sichuan Pepper (Zanthoxylum limonella) oil, one ounce of 100% coconut oil, and three ounces of aloe vera gel. The cost for this recipe is around

$3; that's $2 for the one ounce of Sichuan, and $1 for the coconut oil and aloe vera.

Recipe #8: Use one half ounce of 100% Sichuan Pepper (Zanthoxylum limonella) oil, one half ounce of 100% coconut oil, and four ounces of aloe vera gel. The cost for this recipe is around $2; that's $1 for the one ounce of Sichuan, and $1 for the coconut oil and aloe vera. This is a great budget option. The essential oil component is at 10%, but this level of protection still holds up at 80% effectiveness after 5 hours.

Chapter 4 – Recipes 9-17 Catnip Oil

While there have been a few critics and negative anecdotal discussions against the use of catnip oil, several studies point otherwise. There was an erroneous 2001 study claiming the plant was 10 times as effective as DEET, but that article is suspect. The other thing to keep in mind is that the plant and the essential oil are two separate things. Spreading or rubbing the plant will yield such a small concentration as to be essentially worthless.

In one 2006 study, there was evidence that the catnip essential oil, which contains neptalactone, does in fact provide some protection against mosquitoes, though not quite as much or long as DEET. Still, the catnip essential oil, which can found in 8 ounce bottles at 100% concentration for around $15 dollars is a decent alternative with evidence backing up its usefulness. As such, it's important you know what you are buying. Just having the plant or the leaf is not enough, and you need to make sure you know what is the active ingredients that you are buying. Make sure it is 100% catnip oil with neptalactone, and you can do your own reductions and dilutions for there.

The first few options below combine several active ingredients and essential oils. If I had to pick my favorite recipe, it would be recipe #9. It contains the most effective ingredient, Sichuan, with another tested ingredient, catnip oil, as well as the mustard oil base, with some aloe vera thrown in for good measure. The others that contain catnip oil are good too and great options for those with reactions to Sichuan or mustard oil.

Recipe #9: Use one ounce of 100% Sichuan Pepper (Zanthoxylum limonella) oil and two ounces of 100% Mustard oil as a base. Combine that with .1 ounce of 100% catnip oil (neptalactone), that's .1 ounce not one ounce or about 2 milliliters. Finally add 1.5 ounces of aloe vera. The cost for this recipe is around $11; that's $8 for the catnip oil, $2 for the one ounce of Sichuan, and $1 for the mustard oil & aloe vera. This is the most effective, in my opinion, but it's also the most expensive and smelly.

Recipe #10: Use one ounce of 100% Sichuan Pepper (Zanthoxylum limonella) oil and two ounces of 100% Mustard oil as a base. Combine that with .1 ounces of 100% catnip oil (neptalactone), that's .05 ounce or about 1 milliliter. Finally add 1.5 ounces of aloe vera. The cost for this recipe is around $7; that's $4 for the catnip oil, $2 for the one ounce of Sichuan, and $1 for the mustard oil & aloe vera. This is the second best option for those concerned about price. It maintains the 20% level of essential oils but at a reduced cost.

Recipe #11: Use one half ounce of 100% Sichuan Pepper (Zanthoxylum limonella) oil and one ounce of 100% Mustard oil as a base. Combine that with .1 ounce of 100% catnip oil (neptalactone), that's .05 ounce or about 1 milliliter. Finally add 1.5 ounces of aloe vera. The cost for this recipe is around $6; that's $4 for the catnip oil, $1 for the one ounce of Sichuan, and $1 for the mustard oil & aloe vera. This is still highly effective, but reducing the concentrations of the essential oils to 10% will cut the cost in half and reduce the odor.

Recipe #12: Use one half ounce of 100% Sichuan Pepper (Zanthoxylum limonella) oil, .1 ounces of 100% catnip oil (neptalactone), that's .05 ounce or about 1 milliliter. Finally add 4 ounces of aloe vera. The cost for this recipe is around $6; that's $4 for the catnip oil, $1 for the one ounce of Sichuan, and $1 for the aloe vera. Recipe #12 in similar to #11, holding the concentrations of the essential oils to 10%, but it eliminates the mustard oil for those with reactions. It still includes two great effective ingredients at a reasonable price.

Recipe #13: Use .1 ounce of 100% catnip oil (neptalactone), that's about 2 milliliters. Combine that with 2 ounces of mustard oil. The cost for this recipe is around $9. This recipe is for those with reactions to Sichuan.

Recipe #14: Use one ounce of 100% Sichuan Pepper (Zanthoxylum limonella) oil and two ounces of 100% Coconut oil as a base. Combine that with .1 ounce of 100% catnip oil (neptalactone), that's .1 ounce not one ounce or about 2 milliliters. Finally add 1.5 ounces of aloe vera. The cost for this recipe is around $11; that's $8 for the catnip oil, $2 for the one ounce of Sichuan, and $1 for the coconut oil & aloe vera. This highly effective, but replaces the mustard oil with coconut, a great option for those who don't like the mustard oil base.

Recipe #15: Use one half ounce of 100% Sichuan Pepper (Zanthoxylum limonella) oil and one ounce of 100% coconut oil as a base. Combine that with .1 ounce of 100% catnip oil (neptalactone), that's .05 ounce or about 1 milliliter. Finally add 1.5 ounces of aloe vera. The cost for this recipe is around $6; that's $4 for the catnip oil, $1 for the one ounce of Sichuan, and $1 for the coconut oil & aloe vera. This is still highly effective, but reducing the concentrations of the essential oils to 10% will cut the cost in half and reduce the odor, similar to recipe #10 but with mustard oil instead of coconut oil.

Recipe #16: Use .1 ounce of 100% catnip oil (neptalactone), that's .1 ounces not one ounce or about 2 milliliters. Finally add 1.9 ounces of aloe vera. The cost for this recipe is around $9; that's $8 for the catnip oil, and $1 for the aloe vera. This is a good option for people who cannot tolerate Sichuan, mustard oil, or coconut oil. The 10% concentration of catnip oil is also masked with the aloe vera. This will be less effective than the recipe's with Sichuan, but will work nonetheless.

Keep in mind, though, that this recipe will be effective for a shorter period of time than those without the Sichuan.

Recipe #17: Use .2 ounce (2 mills) of lime oil, one ounce of 100% Sichuan Pepper (Zanthoxylum limonella) oil and two ounces of 100% Mustard oil as a base. Combine that with .1 ounce of 100% catnip oil (neptalactone). Finally, add 1.5 ounces of aloe vera. The cost for this recipe is around $12; that's $8 for the catnip oil, $2 for the one ounce of Sichuan, $2 for the lime oil, and $1 for the mustard oil & aloe vera. This is as effective as as recipe #9 but adds lime oil to the mix. It's one of the more expensive of the recipes, but also the most highly potent. If your skin, nose, and wallet can handle it, this would be a great option.

Chapter 5 – Recipes 18-25

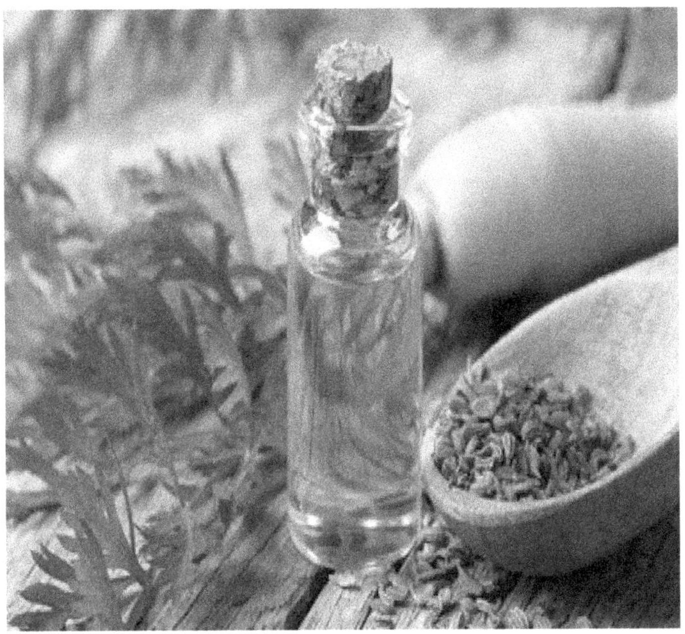

The next set of recipes use the essential oil Lime (Citrus Aurantifolia). As with Sichuan and catnip oil, you want to make sure that the main ingredient is 100% oil and not some watered down derivative. You can find Lime oil at 100% concentrations for about $10 per ounce. This is cheaper than catnip oil but more expensive than Sichuan. Lime oil is also less effective than Sichuan, but still beneficial and a good alternative for those who have reactions to the aforementioned oils.

Recipe #18: Use .5 ounce (10 mills) of lime oil, two ounces of 100% Mustard oil as a base. Combine that with .1 ounce of 100% catnip oil (neptalactone). Finally, add 1.5 ounces of aloe vera. The cost for this recipe is around $14; that's $8 for the catnip oil, $5 for the lime oil, and $1 for the mustard oil & aloe vera. This is as effective as recipe #9 but adds lime oil to the mix. Similar to #17 but without the Sichuan.

Recipe #19: Use .5 ounce (10 mills) of lime oil, two ounces of 100% Coconut oil as a base. Combine that with .1 ounce of 100% catnip oil (neptalactone). Finally, add 1.5 ounces of aloe vera. The cost for this recipe is around $14; that's $8 for the catnip oil, $5 for the lime oil, and $1 for the coconut oil & aloe vera. This is as effective as as recipe #9 but adds lime oil to the mix. Similar to #18 but without replaces the mustard oil with coconut oil and is slightly cheaper.

Recipe #20: Use .5 ounce (10 mills) of lime oil, three ounces of 100% Mustard oil as a base. Finally, add 1.5 ounces of aloe vera. The cost for this recipe is around $6; $5 for the lime oil, and $1 for the mustard oil & aloe vera. This recipe keeps the 20% essential oil threshold but at a lower price.

Recipe #21: Use .3 ounce (10 mills) of lime oil, two ounces of 100% Coconut oil as a base. Finally, add 1 ounces of aloe vera. The cost for this recipe is around $4; $3 for the lime oil, and $1 for the coconut oil & aloe vera. This drops the percentage of essential oil to 10%, but also drops the price, a good budget option.

Recipe #22: Use .2 ounce (10 mills) of lime oil, and 1.8 ounces of aloe vera. The cost for this recipe is around $3; $2 for the lime oil, and $1 for the aloe vera. Recipe #22 is in the cheapest category of all the recipes, but still holds the essential oil to 10%, which hold effectiveness at 80% for up to 5 hours. Great for the budget conscious and also one of the least reactive, so it's great for those with sensitive skin. It's essentially 10% lime oil and 90% aloe vera, simple but effective.

Recipe #23: Use .1 ounce (10 mills) of lime oil, and 1.9 ounces of aloe vera. The cost for this recipe is around $2; $1 for the lime oil, and $1 for the aloe vera. Recipe #22 is in the cheapest category of all the recipes and drops the essential oil to 5%, which hold effectiveness at 60-70% for up to 5 hours. This may be a decent option for the budget minded and those with extremely sensitive skin. The simple basic components are 5% lime oil and 95% aloe vera.

Recipe #24: Use .2 ounce (10 mills) of lime oil, and 1.8 ounces of 100% agave nectar. The cost for this recipe is around $3; $2 for the lime oil, and $1 for the agave nectar. Recipe #24 is simple and cheap. A great option with the added moisturizing effects of agave, and it still holds the essential oil to 10%, which hold effectiveness at 80% for up to 5 hours.

Recipe #25: our final recipe, uses .1 ounce (10 mills) of lime oil, and 1.9 ounces of agave nectar. Like recipe #22, it's tied for the cheapest recipe and drops the essential oil to 5%, which hold effectiveness at 60-70% for up to 5 hours. This may be a good option for the budget minded and those with extremely sensitive skin. If you prefer agave nectar to aloe, and you have sensitive skin, this final option may be for you.

When looking at all the 25 recipes listed above, feel free to switch the filler ingredients for something else you prefer and change the concentrations to your liking. Just remember, for maximum effectiveness you want the essential oil to be in the 10-20% concentration range or greater in a mustard base. Drop the concentration no lower than 5% for sensitive skin, and keep any swamped ingredients to those with minimal or no scent.

Conclusion

The world of simplifying, prepping, and getting closer to nature no longer has to
be fraught with an attack of the killer mosquitoes. While you can't eliminate

yourself completely as a target, it's easier than ever to safeguard both your home and your body from these nasty and dangerous pests. Remember that most other remedies that target eliminated mosquitoes are ineffective or worse. Much of your preparation will involve simple basic steps that reduce the opportunity for mosquitoes to breed. Also, make sure that you still follow common sense steps to reduce your risk of being bitten, such as staying dry, cool, and covered; and when you make your repellent, don't forget to include 10% or more of the studied essential oils to maximize its effectiveness.

Don't let this book be something you read and forget. Take the easy steps necessary to put into place the simple solutions of making do it yourself repellent before you become the latest victim of one of the slew of mosquito borne illnesses that are ravaging the globe. Enjoy the great outdoors, but enjoy it safely.

FREE Bonus Reminder

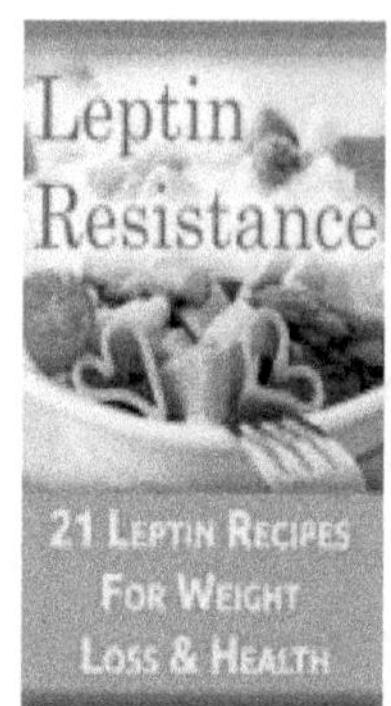

If you have not grabbed it yet, please go ahead and download your special bonus report *"Leptin Resistance. 21 Leptin Recipes For Weight Loss & Healthy Living"*.

Simply Click the Button Below

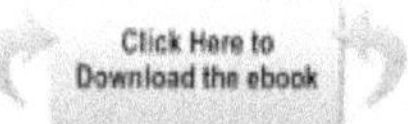

OR **Go to This Page**

http://easyweightlossway.com/free/

BONUS #2: More Free & Discounted Books

Do you want to receive more Free & Discounted Books?

We have a mailing list where we send out our new Books when they go free or with a discount on Kindle. Click on the link below to sign up for Free & Discount Book Promotions.

=> Sign Up for Free & Discount Book Promotions <=

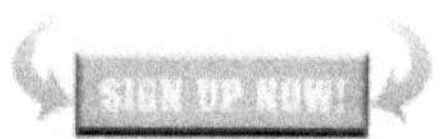

OR Go to this URL

http://zbit.ly/1WBb1Ek